NUTRITION 101

Nutrition Basics and implementation

Mariana Molinari-Abadie

Strength Sisters 101

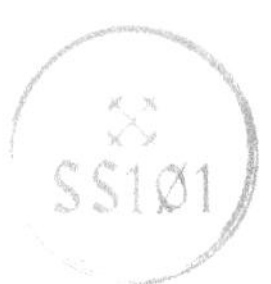

Strength TRAINING 101
~Nutrition Edition~

1- Basic Nutrition

Flexible diet, Calories, macro, and micronutrient requirements.

Which method is best for you?

2- Calorie counting

Basic needs, deficiencies, supplements.

Important considerations before you start.

Tracking, Adjusting, Competent, Intuitive.

3- Habits and skills vs. dieting

Habits to master, building skills until they become habits.

4- Metabolism

NEAT, Stress, Sleep, Night Shift Workers, Injury Recovery.

5- Facts that may help you reach your goals easier

Good carbs, bad carbs (no such thing), and the humble potato.

Breaking out with fad diets.

Carbs; why do some people fear them and others love them?

Links and References.

1- Basic Nutrition

Macro and Micronutrient Requirements

Protein, carbs, fats, fiber. Phytonutrients. Essential amino acids.

"The food we eat is composed of a variety of nutrients. As the chemical structures of these nutrients are fairly large, we must break them down into smaller, unbound, more soluble units in order to be absorbed into the body. Once absorbed, these smaller units become usable by our cell, and once they enter the general circulation, their actual food source doesn't really matter; once broken down and absorbed, the body doesn't necessarily recognize the difference between the amino acids derived from whey protein in the form of protein powder or the ones derived from milk. Nor does it recognize the difference between glucose derived from whole wheat bread or the one from table sugar. And it doesn't recognize the difference between monounsaturated fats from a hamburger or monounsaturated fats from olive oil. (Excerpt from The essentials of sport and exercise nutrition, PN)

The difference is in the nutrients they deliver, so you do want some fruits and vegetables for fiber, vitamins, minerals, and phytosterols but other than that, it doesn't matter where your carbs are coming from once you met nutrition needs, that's why the 80% whole foods and 20%

whatever you want works well.

Calories

What is a calorie?

A calorie is a unit of measure that indicates the amount of energy we obtain from a particular food.

The scientific definition of a calorie, is the amount of energy, or heat, it takes to raise the temperature of 1 gram of water 1 degree Celsius.

Macronutrients

The foods we eat contain one or a combination of the three macronutrients: protein, fat, and carbohydrates. Each macronutrient has a caloric value. Carbohydrates and Proteins are 4 calories per gram, and Fat has 9 calories per gram. Alcohol has about 7 calories per gram but is not considered a macronutrient, it is considered a toxin. Our body uses each macronutrient for different processes, which means that tracking your intake has a profound effect on factors such as body composition, energy availability, performance, mood, and general well-being. We store body fat by consuming more total calories than our bodies use or burn. No single macronutrient is responsible for fat loss.

PROTEIN

Protein is used as the building block for almost every tissue in our body, so consuming enough quality protein is essential for repairing, building, and optimal function. The amount required is dependent on many factors such as your body composition goals, age, level of leanness, and dietary history among others.

The body has the ability to make 12 amino acids, known as non-essential amino acids. However, 8 amino acids can only be supplied by the diet and are thus termed essential amino acids. Hence the importance of daily amino acid intake through the food we consume. Small daily losses from amino acid breakdown will eventually put us in a net negative protein balance. While carbohydrate and especially fat content of the body is fairly well maintained, it's actually quite difficult to maintain a consistent amino acid pool without dietary intervention. Managing the plasma amino acid pool is like keeping a sink full without a drain plug. If amino acid intake falls below daily amino acid degradation, things like enzymes and structural proteins are cannibalized. If this process persists for long enough, vital functions shut down. As for protein quality, animal proteins such as meat, poultry, eggs, fish, milk, and cheese, rank the highest while plant proteins rank lower. (Extracted from The Essentials of Sport and Exercise Nutrition-PN).

While not every protein source you eat needs to be complete, ensure that the proteins you eat provide the necessary combination of amino acids for your body to repair and grow muscle adequately. This is the main reason why if you consume enough quality source protein, BCAAs are useless.

Some examples of **complete** proteins are: ◉ Meat ◉ Poultry ◉ Fish ◉ Eggs ◉ Dairy (whey protein, Greek yogurt) ◉ Soy ◉ Spirulina ◉ Quinoa

Some examples of foods containing **incomplete** proteins are: ◉ Vegetables ◉ Seeds and nuts (nut butter) ◉ Legumes ◉ Grains

CARBOHYDRATES

There's a debate whether carbohydrates are essential or not, but even though our bodies can function without them, it is far from optimal.

Carbs are used as the main source of energy by the body, brain, liver, to make glycogen, etc.

Also, without carb sources such as fruits and vegetables, we'd be missing important micronutrients, vitamins, minerals, phytosterols, fiber... which contribute to our optimal performance and well-being. Fiber is important for proper digestion; contains prebiotics which is the fiber our friendly bacteria (probiotics) eat, hence optimal for gut health.

Examples of foods that are primarily carbohydrates include: ◉ Fruits ◉Vegetables ◉ Grains ◉ Potatoes ◉ Rice, pasta ◉ Honey, sugars

FATS

Fats are an essential macronutrient; our body can't function without enough essential fatty acids coming from foods. Adequate intake of dietary fats is important for proper hormone function, proper fat-soluble vitamin absorption, to synthesize cholesterol, and also as a stored source of energy for long-lasting activities such as distance running or other low to medium intensity long-lasting cardiovascular activities.

Some fats are healthier than others. Among the different types of dietary fat, we find Saturated, Monounsaturated, and Polyunsaturated (omega-3 and 6), and Trans-Fats. Trans fats are the only ones that should be avoided altogether since they are harmful. Saturated fats should be limited since they may have some negative health effects if consumed in excess, but they may even have benefits when consumed in moderation. Polyunsaturated fats are essential for life and health, and monounsaturated fats are beneficial as well.

Examples of trans fats (avoid): ◉ Hydrogenated and partially hydrogenated vegetable oil ◉ Shortening ◉ Some margarine products ◉ In many ultra-processed foods

Examples of saturated fats (moderate): ◉ Coconut oil/palm oil ◉ Animal fats (from meat) ◉ Butter

Examples of polyunsaturated fats (essential): ◉ Fish oil ◉ Nuts/ Seeds ◉ Some plant-based oils such as sunflower oil

Examples of monounsaturated fats: ◉ Avocado/Avocado oil ◉ Grapeseed oil ◉ Olive oil ◉ Canola oil

2- Calorie counting, basic needs, deficiencies, supplements

CALORIC ESTIMATION

Counting calories; I personally don't think that counting is something to adopt as an everyday thing or a habit, but it's a very useful tool and gives us a good idea of our general nutrient intake. It's a resource that can be used as needed. And it is easier than it seems.

So, first and foremost, let's make these basics of calorie counting very clear:

Perfection is not possible because inaccuracies in counting are unavoidable.

Simplifications make life easier, but we introduce an additional layer of inaccuracy.

Inaccuracies (to a degree) are fine as long as we are consistently inaccurate – we can then make relative adjustments to our intake after a baseline has been established over several weeks of consistency.

When counting calories, we need to know how many calories our body needs according to our activity level, diet history, age, type of diet, etc. it is different for everybody, so finding your own needs is imperative to achieve results. That's why celebrity XYZ's latest 1,200 calorie diet won't work for anyone long term nor for anyone with different needs and might actually be detrimental to health and performance.

A most accurate way to find your maintenance calories

If your weight is stable, you are eating at caloric balance, so for the first week, don't introduce any changes to your diet, just record the calories from your usual intake. At the end of the week take the mean (average) from those numbers (sum all the results from each day and divide by the number of days, 7 if a week) to get your average intake or maintenance calories.

So, for the second week, take that average number and deduct around 200/500 cal for weight loss or add them for weight gain. Repeat the counting process and record if you notice any weight changes. Slim individuals should aim for the smallest deficit possible and consume enough protein to prevent muscle loss in the process.

If your weight decreased, you are at a caloric deficit, if your weight increased, you are at a surplus and if you remained the same, you are still at balance, often due to miscalculations, decreased in NEAT (Non-exercise activity thermogenesis), or masked by water retention, etc. (More on NEAT later).

Now, according to your results, you can either lower calorie intake (~10% total calories) or increase (~10% total calories) or keep them the same, depending on if you are trying to lose weight or gain weight and you are not on track with reaching those goals with your current intake. About 1% body weight loss/gain seems like a healthy guideline to follow, of course, you can lose faster or slower, but there is a risk of losing lean body mass (muscle) while on a deficit or gain more fat than desired when bulking. You can also modify caloric balance with more or less exercise/movement, but generally, exercise won't make a big impact unless you are a professional athlete or have a very active demanding job.

A less accurate method would be to start at an estimated caloric and macronutrient value and adjust from what you see happening in the next couple of weeks.

How to calculate your MACROS

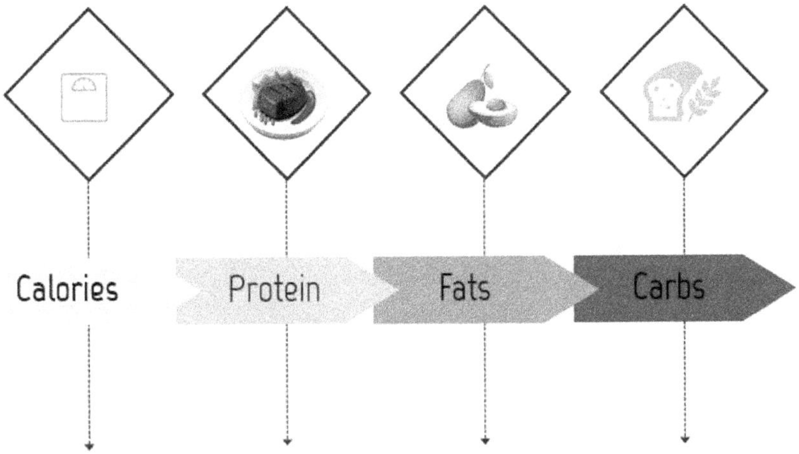

Calories	Protein	Fats	Carbs

Calculate your dieting Calories

Multiply your bodyweight in pounds by 10-12 according to activity level.

Higher activity higher end.

(x 14-16 for maintenance).

Calculate Protein

Multiply your bodyweight 0.8-1.2 for protein grams.

(Higher end the leaner you are).

Multiply x 4 for **Protein** calories.

Calculate Fat

Multiply your bodyweight x 0.25-0.4 for fat grams.

Multiply x 9 for **Fat** calories.

Calculate Carbs

Substract protein and fat calories from your dieting calories for carb calories.

Divide your carb calories by 4 for **carb** grams.

Strength Sisters 101

BASIC ESTIMATIONS:

Multiplying your body weight in pounds by (10x your bodyweight) is as close to your BMR (Basal Metabolic Rate = The calories your body needs to repair itself without any movement) as it gets; 12x your bodyweight gives you a safe range of calories to lose weight; 13-14x bodyweight is usually close to maintenance for most people, and 15-16x or more is for gaining.

Activity level is adjusted and accounted for in these calculations, less active people would use the lower end, and more active the higher end of those calculations. When very overweight or obese your calculations may be even lower than the average due to body composition, but not always.

Protein:

After finding the optimal caloric needs according to your goal, we have to find adequate protein intake for your goal, muscle preservation, or building taking into consideration dietary habits (vegetarians need more protein due to the quality of the protein ingested which is mostly coming from non-complete sources).

Protein requirement is not a number set in stone, it depends on several variables including quality of protein ingested, age, fitness level, and of course, individual repair needs. The recommended minimum for sedentary individuals is 0.8g/Kg, this translates to about 55g of protein per day for a 150lb individual. However, this amount is not optimal but simply to prevent protein deficiency. During high-intensity training, these needs may be increased to about 1.4 to 2.0g per Kg of body mass (between 95 and 135g of protein per day for a 150lb individual). Similar increases are recommended during periods of low energy intake or low carbohydrate intake.

When attempting to build muscle or retain muscle mass in a caloric deficit, the amount needed is much higher than the minimum amount needed for basic health or avoiding deficiency. Basic guidelines for improving body composition is a range, from .8g-1.5g per lb of total body weight. Less is needed in a calorie surplus, while more is needed (for muscle preservation) in a calorie deficit. Obese individuals may go as low as .7g per lb of total body weight. Adjust your protein requirements accordingly. Keep in mind that as you lose weight, you should increase protein requirements if you attempt to get leaner.

Fats:

Now we figure out essential fatty acids (Fats): Even though there is a minimum amount of dietary fat required for optimal health, there isn't enough research for a certain amount to be known. It is stipulated that around 0.35 g per lb of bodyweight give or take preference is a safe place to calculate.

Carbohydrates:

Keep in mind that fats are 9 calories per gram while carbs are only 4 calories per gram, so as you calculate this out of preference, carbs will give you more volume of foods than fats. It is also important that your diet contains enough carbs to fuel your activity level. Sedentary individuals need fewer carbs, while those exercising hard need more for proper performance. If carbs are too low, you may feel lethargic, tired, ending in poor performance which in turn will burn fewer calories, decrease your NEAT and provide less stimulus during your workouts being detrimental for muscle building or fat loss.

Fiber (optional):

Other than Protein, Fats, and Carbs, you may want to track fiber to make sure you are getting enough. Fibrous foods may help with satiety, keeping you feeling fuller for longer. The Academy of Nutrition and Dietetics recommends approximately 14 grams of fiber for every 1000 calories consumed.

Sugar, Salt, Others:

Some trackers prompt you to track sugars or salt but unless you have a specific condition that requires you to consume low sugar or salt, there is no need to track them separately. Make sure you track total carbs and not "net carbs" which is only meaningful for diabetics or people with specific metabolic conditions that need to track them.

When you are attempting a caloric deficit or controlling calories, it is important to focus on consuming more volume of foods and not less to prevent hunger, adding foods that are satiating and bulky can go a long way. Also, hydrating properly can help. Keep in mind that fats are very caloric dense, meaning that a little miscalculation can quickly put you over your calorie allotment. Protein and carbs are 4 calories per gram and fats are 9 calories per gram. Potatoes are the most satiating food as long as you don't add oils or dressing to them, use them when hungry, an apple before meals can help with hunger too. Spinach may help with energy.

When bulking or looking to gain mass, you are not at risk of losing muscle mass as it happens when we are in a caloric deficit, so you don't even need to worry much about a lot of protein, your body won't be consuming muscle for energy if you are NOT in a deficit. Still make sure you get enough basic nutrition for proper performance, repair, and growth, meaning most of your foods coming from whole sources, protein (not necessarily from lean sources), vegetables but once the basics are met, you can play with adding high caloric foods such as ice cream, nut butter, nuts, seeds, avocado, oils, granola, whole dairy, chocolate, and anything you like if your calories aren't met.

NO MATTER YOUR GOAL, FOCUS ON THE MOST IMPORTANT BLOCKS FIRST

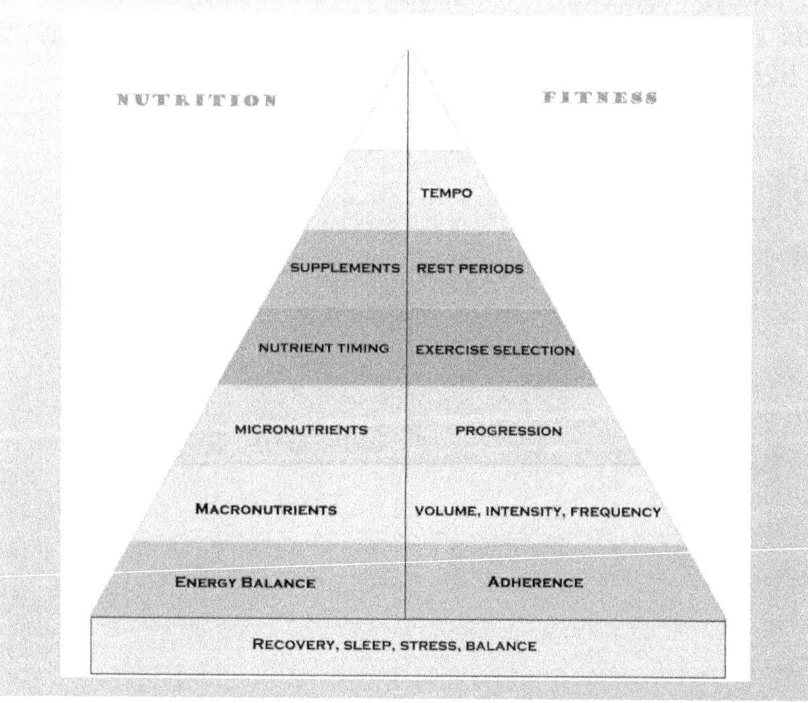

Energy (caloric) Balance. Food composition. Nutrients, Macro & Micro Nutrients. Repair, Recovery, Build, Sleep, Stress. Variety, the dose makes the poison, anti-nutrients (phytic acid), absorption. Nutrient timing, Hydration, Supplements.

Calorie Cycling

For anyone attempting a caloric deficit no matter the medium, keep in mind that our bodies do not work on a daily schedule but on a time period, whether that is a day, a week, or a month. So, a caloric deficit can be attempted for a few days, a week, a month, etc. One day of a higher caloric intake is, therefore, not a failure, it can be perfectly included and even planned in a weekly/monthly deficit.

Any strict regimen consisting of low calories or low carbohydrates can be very taxing, not only to our body but also to our mind, especially over a long-term period.

Restricting calories and/or carbohydrates for long periods can have negative metabolic effects, so it's important to plan and manipulate intake to make it easier, sustainable, and less stressful on both, mind and body.

For example, if you cycle days of lower and days of higher calories, you can give yourself a day break when you need it most; those days can be planned or forgiven if you happen to increase calories by accident one day, it's O.K. to allow enough wiggle room when needed to help with adherence and sanity.

A good idea is to keep protein and fat intake relatively constant while carbohydrate intake is manipulated because higher carbohydrate intake days can increase thyroid output and control hunger, they are also a great energy source on workout days.

It doesn't matter when or where you include those higher days or if they happen by accident, if the overall long-term trend is towards a negative energy balance, you can have your cake and eat it too.

Calorie Cycling

CONSTANT CALORIES

Monday	Tuesday	Wednesday	Thursday	Friday	Saturday	Sunday	
1500	1500	1500	1500	1500	1500	1500	**Weekly average 1500**

HIGHER CALORIES ON WORKOUT DAYS

Monday	Tuesday	Wednesday	Thursday	Friday	Saturday	Sunday	
1600	1350	1600	1350	1600	1500	1500	**Weekly average 1500**

HIGHER CALORIES ON WEEKEND

Monday	Tuesday	Wednesday	Thursday	Friday	Saturday	Sunday	
1400	1400	1400	1400	1750	1750	1400	**Weekly average 1500**

Supplementing from food deficiency

Some supplements are essential nutrients that come from the food we eat because they can not be made by the body, these ones can also be supplemented if we aren't consuming the adequate amount in our diet, they can be used regularly or occasionally depending on individual needs (fish oil, multivitamins, Vit D in some cases, protein, and even greens and recovery drinks), these are essential and need supplementation when they are NOT being met by the diet or in some special occasions as recovery drinks for elite athletes, marathon runners, etc. Also, when in a caloric deficit or special diets (vegans, etc.) it is more of an umbrella policy to cover what may be missed by restricting calories. Then, we have the non-essential supplements which may be beneficial in certain situations, but many are unlikely to make a difference in recreational athletes, this is where creatine, caffeine, EGCG, and others that are very case-specific come in, like melatonin, or the right combination of magnesium+zinc right before sleeping for relaxation.

Adequate intake from food and/or supplements is necessary to prevent deficiency, so, it is important to recognize the symptoms of those deficiencies as well as what we may be missing depending on the composition of our diet (restricting, vegan, carnivore, etc.), to adjust when necessary through food or supplementation.

Where do I find the macronutrient I need?

Here is a convenient macronutrients list:

Foods and their Macronutrients.

Strength Sisters 101

NEED CARBS + FATS

Fruit & Nuts	Nut butter fudge	Coconut flakes	Buttery popcorn
Nut butter & Fruit	Avocado toast	Cookies	Dried fruit & nuts
Chocolate	Donuts	Potato chips	Flavored whole milk
Seeds/Chia	French fries	Tortilla chips	Chocolate coverd fruit/nuts

HIGH VOLUME LOW MACROS

SNACKS
Plain Popcorn
Seaweed
Sugar free jello
Rice cakes
Cucumber
Celery
Skinny noodles

FRUITS/VEGGIES
Carrots
Cucumbers
Celery
Cabbage
Lettuce
Cauliflower
Broccoli
Pickles
Mushrooms
Strawberries
Lemon/Lime
Sprouts
Radishes

BEVERAGES
Water/Sparkling
Hot/iced tea
Hot/iced Coffee
Zero sodas
Zero waters
Skimmed broth
Low cal milks
Artificial sweets
Aspartame/Stevia

CONDIMENTS
Vinegar
Lenon/Lime
Light Mayo
Mustard
Smoke flavor
Hot sauce
Salsa
Sriracha
Horseradish
Pickles
Nonfat yogurt
PB2
Calorie free syrup
100% Cocoa
Ranch packets

CARBOHYDRATES

Fruits/Dried fruit
Potatoes/Sweetpotato
Squash/Pumpkin
Root vegetables
Rice/Pasta
Grains/Cereals
Honey/Syrup
Corn tortillas
Flour tortillas
Jam/Jelly
Popcorn plain
Candy/Gummies
Balsamic vinegar
Tomato souce/Ketchup
Barbecue sauce
Flours in general
Juice/Soda
Sugary drinks
Sugar/Nectar
Rice cakes

PROTEIN

Lean meats
Deli meat
Whey protein
Soy protein
Egg whites
Chicken breast skinless
Pork tenderloin
Lean turkey
Shrimp
Non fatty fish
Tuna/Cod/Flounder
Fat free cotagge cheese
Nonfat Greek yogurt
Nonfat ricotta

Vegetarian seitan
Firm tofu
Black bean paste

FATS

Avocado
Olives'
Olive Oil
Vegetable oil
Chicken/pork skin
Nut butter
Peanut/almond butter
Nuts/seeds
Mayonnaise
Walnuts/Macadamia
Sunflower seeds/Chia
Fish oil
Flaxseeds/Hempseeds
Salad dressing
Butter/Margarine
90% dark chocolate
Nut flour/Almond
Almond butter
Full fat dairy/Cheese
Bone marrow

CARBOHYDRATES + PROTEIN

Fat free flavored Greek yogurt
Fat free flavored milk
Cereal+skim milk
Oats+Whey
Plain Greek yogurt+fruit
Crackers+Deli meat
Sandwich (Plain bread/Meat/chiken)
Potatoes & egg whites
Lean fish & rice
Tuna wrap
Whole wheat bread+deli meat
Veggies+Egg whites
Fruit sprikled with whey
Fruit/whey smoothie
Overnight oats (fruit/yogurt/whey)
Cereal+whey shake
Veggie omelette (egg whites only)
Tuna+Ketchup
Veggies with Greek yogurt dip

FATS + PROTEIN

Cheeses/full fat dairy
Hummus
Nut butters
Nuts
Avocado+Smoked salmon
Fatty cuts of meat/Pork
Chicken with skin
Cotagge cheese full fat
Greek yogurt whole milk
Sour cream
Protein shake with peanut butter
Sausage/Brats
Chicken thighs/Turkey dark
Salmon/Fatty fish
Fried eggs
Coconut milk+protein shake
Most jerky
Eggs
High fat Ground beef/pork

Important considerations before you start

When weighing your foods, you have to make sure you weigh everything you taste, including liquids (unless it is calorie-free like water or plain tea or coffee) even if it is only a sip or to taste the food you are cooking or someone else's food, etc. Liquids aren't only drinks, it's cooking oils, dressings, etc. EVERYTHING that goes in needs to be weighed in its original state (most foods like they come in their packaging, rice and pasta uncooked, meats raw, etc.)

And you don't have to be meticulous about it forever, but for awareness and learning purposes it is important to do it right for some time until you know the portions and actual calories of those portions.

MFP is a good tracking tool if you know how to properly measure and track and if you use it responsibly for a short time, but it is not good for calculating your caloric needs.

Most other tracking apps have issues of their own so it's very important to learn how to measure properly. When you are eating in a surplus this doesn't matter much; at maintenance, you can be a little sloppy but when cutting this becomes extremely important.

Also, be careful with My Fitness Pal and other trackers, make sure to not allow the "calories burned" to be added as extra calories you can consume because they should not be eaten back.

Keep in mind that obsessively tracking can cause eating disorder behaviors such as binge/restrict cycles, stop if you see this happening (PLEASE!). It is also OK to stop and take breaks at maintenance when needed but one meal or one day a week of overeating may be undoing the weekly deficit if it is not tracked and accounted for, it's OK to plan a higher intake one day or meal a week but you have to still track it an make sure that is not as high in calories as to undo the weekly deficit.

Tracking can be a very helpful tool for awareness purposes but it shouldn't be used in the long term. Learning to eat mindfully along the way according to the portions we see when we measure is a good way to move into a more intuitive or competent way of eating.

Moving from tracking everything to "intuitive eating" is also a learning experience that I like to call competent eating; the maintenance phase can be the most challenging because most people left to intuition, they'll overeat or miss some much-needed nutrients, and to be able to eat without overdoing it, we have to learn a set of skills that may come from counting, portioning, or satiating cues or a mix of all of them. If you've been counting, you can probably guess how hungry you feel once your calories/macros are met. Depending on what you have been consuming, you can probably guess that if you add a specific treat one day, you'll end up your day with not enough calories left to satiate your hunger cues and if you've been adding enough protein and bulk (vegetables/fiber) to your meals, you are probably going to be satisfied by the end of the day. It takes a bit of paying attention to that while you are counting or portioning or learning habits until they go in autopilot because they become your way of eating, that's competent eating when you can be trusted to make the choices that will give your body the nutrition it needs without measuring everything and only go back to counting if you see some deviations from what you are expecting.

3- Habits and skills vs. dieting

This section is dedicated to all of you that have tried it all but still feel that are struggling, to the chronic dieters that feel like nothing works for them, to those that are starting to understand that quick fixes don't work but they do not know what else to do, because let me tell you, it's not you and it's not your fault. We've been misled by the media and the gurus that want to profit from our lack of results in the long term so they can keep selling us more quick fixes, diet books, and miracle pills.

There is no one way to do things and not a single way will work for everyone. You've probably heard before that diets don't work, yet everyone keeps doing them and they seem to work for them, at least for a while, and that's where the problem is, anyone can lose weight if they find a way to reduce caloric intake no matter what they do to achieve that caloric imbalance, consume fewer calories than you burn and voila, results start happening. Except that those results are usually short-lived. Sometimes because those diets aren't sustainable and as soon as the previous behaviors are resumed, they stop working and weight is regained, other times because restriction causes neverending binge/restrict cycles, and sometimes, they plain end up spiraling into unhealthy behaviors.

So, what work do you say? What seems to work well, is creating habits by changing behaviors that will last a lifetime instead of short-lived quick fixes that don't solve anything in the long run and more often than not, may end up being counterproductive or unhealthy.

The key is to take one single behavior at a time and work on it to make it into a habit, and only once this habit becomes so ingrained in you that you don't have to think about doing it anymore, is that you can introduce another behavior to change and form into another habit. This last step is very important because when we try to change many things at once, none will stick, and guess what? It is not your fault, it is part of human behavior.

This is going to be long but worth the read. It is an excerpt from the book "The Power of Less". Hope it helps

"Give out one clear task, and 85% of clients can stick to it. Add a second task, and adherence drops to less than 35%. Three tasks – pfft. Now you've got less than 10% success." So start with one habit; ideally, a habit that's small, manageable, and as practical as possible. When in doubt, simply take your one assigned task and reduce the difficulty by half.

This is the main idea:

1-Select one habit...only one habit per month (ideally one habit for two months). You can choose any habit – whatever you think will have the biggest impact on your life.

2-Write down your plan. You will need to specifically state what your goal will be each day, when you'll do it, what your "trigger" will be, who you will report to...

3-Post your goal publicly. Tell as many people as possible that you are trying to form your new habit. I suggest an online forum, but you could email it to coworkers and family and friends or otherwise get the word out to a large group.

4-Report on your progress daily. Each day, tell the same group of people whether or not you succeeded at your goal."

There are only a few rules you need to follow to make this challenge a success:

-Do only one habit at a time. Do not break this rule, because I assure you that if you do multiple habits at once, you will be much less likely to succeed. Trust me

– I've tried both ways many times, and in my experience, there is 100% failure for forming multiple habits at once, and a 50-80% success if you do just one habit at a time – depending on whether you follow the rest of these rules.

-Choose an easy goal (behavior). Don't decide to do something really hard, at least for now. Later, when you're good at habit changes, you can choose something harder. But for now, do something you know you can do every day. In fact, choose something easier than you think you can do every day. If you think you can exercise for 30 minutes a day, choose 10 minutes – making it super easy is one of the surest ways to ensure you'll succeed.

-Choose something measurable. You should be able to say, definitively, whether you were successful or not today. If you choose to exercise, set a number of minutes or something similar (20 minutes of exercise daily, for example). Whatever your goal, have a measurement.

-Be consistent. You want to do your habit change at the same time every day, if possible. If you're going to exercise, do it at 7 a.m. (or 6 p.m.) every day, for example. This makes it more likely to become a habit.

-Report daily. You could check in every 2 or 3 days, but you'll be more likely to succeed if you report daily. This has been proven over and over again.

-Expect setbacks now and then, but just note them and move on. No embarrassment, no failures."

There are many habits or strategies that you can pick, (portion control, working on the skills needed to eating mindfully until full, add protein to every meal, add vegetables to each meal, move more, walk daily, etc.) but trying them all together is usually overwhelming and why it seems unrealistic, unsustainable and ends up not working.

Just one simple change practiced over the course of a few months makes a lifetime of difference. Then we can reevaluate and see if there is a need/want to add any other habit that can enrich our lives that we may want to work on.

See if this is something that may work for you, otherwise, as I said before, there are many ways or paths that can lead to where we want to go, we just have to find one that we are comfortable with according to our own preferences and lifestyle.

Beginners with modest goals with simple basic steps looking to improve overall health:

If your aim is fat loss, you should be looking at habits that will reduce your caloric intake or increase your caloric expenditure by moving more, a combination of both is recommended.

A variety of foods that you enjoy usually works best for accountability and sustainability, aim for 80% whole foods and 20% of what your soul desires.

Try to pick one habit at a time and stick with it for at least 2 months before adding another one. Once that first habit becomes part of your daily routine, then you can add a second habit.

These simple habits can often help you do that without counting calories.

Habits to master:

1- Eat mindfully and make sure to stop at 80% full.

Relax and take your time to enjoy your food and check with hunger frequently.

Make sure to stop eating when you're about 80% full.

2- Eat protein-dense foods with each meal.

Try to aim for at least 1 palm-size portion of protein with every meal.

3- Vegetables with every meal.

Add vegetables to every meal. 1 fist-size is a portion, you can eat as many portions as you like with each meal.

4-Carbs.

Smaller portions of starchy carbs and larger of vegetables with meals and majority of starchy carbs around workouts/exercise.

Again as many vegetables as you want.

(Be careful with dressings, they do not count as vegetables and are often loaded with extra calories)

5-Eat healthy fats daily.

Prioritize fats from whole sources like eggs, meat, fish, nuts, seeds, olives.

You can add Omega fish oil supplement.

Last but not least:

If you reduce your caloric intake it is not a bad idea to take a daily multivitamin supplement to make sure your micro-nutrients are covered.

Focus on rewarding habits instead of outcomes, some of these habits take a bit of time to kick in. See, "I need to lose 10 pounds" is an outcome, "I need to exercise five times per week" is a behavior; followed this week's habits 90% of the time and didn't miss any workouts? That's worthy of a reward regardless of the outcome because it's this pattern of behavior that will eventually lead to success.

If instead of working with habits you'd rather count calories, I'll put all that together in the next section, how to figure out your caloric balance, how to increase or decrease depending on your goals, etc.

Even if you reduce your caloric intake and you are achieving results from eating habits alone, it's always a good idea to add movement, any kind of movement counts, even fidgeting adds up to your calorie expenditure and moving has lots of benefits for overall health.

4- Metabolism, NEAT, Stress, Sleep, Injury Recovery

NEAT (Non-Exercise Activity Thermogenesis).

METABOLISM – BMR (Basal Metabolic Rate) -TEF (Thermic Effect of Food) – EEE Exercise Energy Expenditure) – NEAT (Non-Exercise Activity Thermogenesis).

Do you know why increasing cardio is not giving you the expected results? That's because, during a caloric deficit, the physical activity components, Exercise and NEAT, of the calorie equation are indirectly proportional to each other, the more exercise you do, the more your body will conserve energy and decrease NEAT (fidgeting, pacing, and overall desire to move).

BMR or Basal/Resting Metabolic Rate: Energy essential to maintain your body functioning.

TEF or Thermic Effect of Food: Energy utilized to break down and digest the food.

EEE or Exercise Energy Expenditure: Extra energy that is spent through intentional exercise.

NEAT or Non-Exercise Activity Thermogenesis: Energy that you burn while moving around during the day that is not intentional exercise (pacing, fidgeting, bouncing, etc.)

This is how much each influence what we call metabolism:

BMR: 50-60%

TEF: ~10%

EEE: ~5-15%

NEAT: ~20%

As we can clearly see, the function that consumes the most calories is our resting metabolic rate and the one that can make a difference along the day would be NEAT. But our BMR seems to be the most important aspect, studies have shown that even when someone has a slower metabolism than normal, the variants aren't large and it has minimal influence on weight loss/gain. That's why, when calculating your BMR, a little miscalculation won't make a large difference (~50/100 calories).

When we look at NEAT, that's a different story because the difference in NEAT among people can be very high, a lot higher than a mere 50/100 calories from BMR. Depending on weight, height, age, and other factors, NEAT can vary ~1000 calories from person to person.

What is NEAT?

NEAT (Non-Exercise Activity Thermogenesis) Adaptations

Probably the most significant adaptation to weight changes is in NEAT

With weight loss, your body burns fewer calories doing your usual daily chores such as pacing or fidgeting; it also decreases your motivation to conciously and subconciously move.

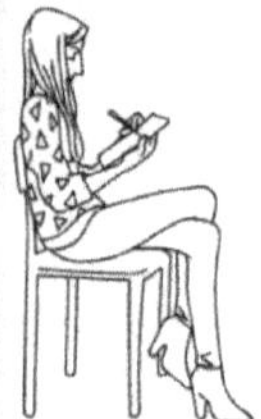
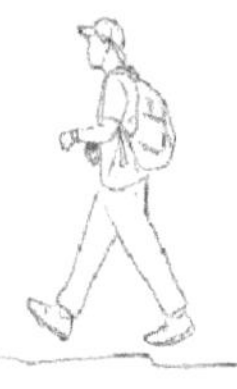
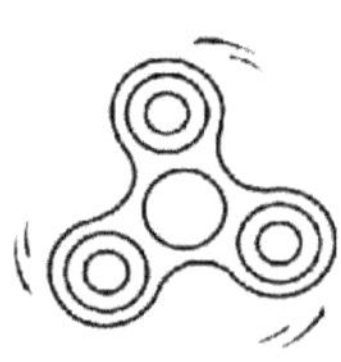

| More Sitting | Less Pacing/Walking | Less Fidgeting | Less Overall Calories Burned |

But, we have to be careful because EEE and NEAT are indirectly proportional to each other, the more exercise you do, the more your body will conserve energy and decrease NEAT, and too much intentional cardio will eventually interfere with recovery as well.

As coaches, we monitor recovery and energy/fatigue feelings weekly or on the daily in some cases to adjust these important factors because more is not always better. Strategically increasing or decreasing your NEAT intentionally depending on your goals may make a difference that worrying about your BMR or counting calories to perfection may not.

The Role of Non-exercise Activity Thermogenesis in Human Obesity:
https://www.ncbi.nlm.nih.gov/books/NBK279077/?
fbclid=IwAR1L-9qA1QuyVbqpseI4VsKxtN0jWt0i44CEGSmHcpyBgHC7Z51JhB_sLxA

Total Energy Expenditure

During a caloric deficit, the physical activity components, Exercise and NEAT, of the calorie equation are indirectly proportional to each other, the more exercise you do, the more your body will conserve energy and decrease NEAT (fidgeting, pacing, and overall desire to move).

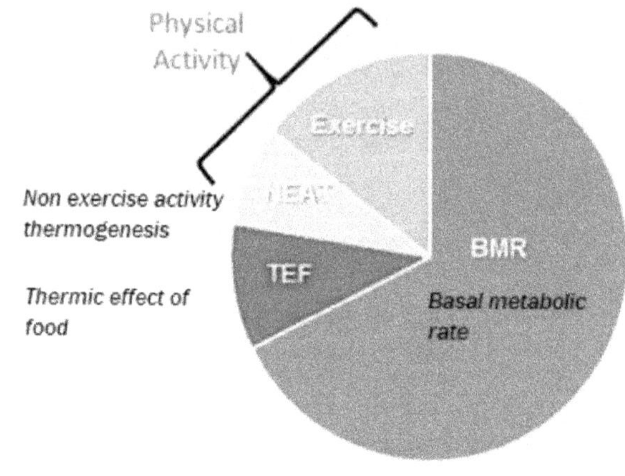

STRESS:

Stress is very taxing, whether it is imposed through exercise, or coming from work, family, lack of sleep, etc. without enough recovery, training instead of building you, it can break you down and you'll end with a recovery debt that can lead to injuries, constant pain, chronic fatigue, etc. Try to balance exercise with the rest of your life's happenings while you can enjoy what you are doing. There are days where stress might come from non-exercise sources but we still need recovery.

If you are training intensely multiple times per week and have a full-time job and a family, stressors are acting upon you in all directions. Without proper planning, training will no longer serve as a catalyst to meet your physical goals; it'll break you down. And contrary to popular thinking, the more your training evolves, the more stress you impose on yourself. An intermediate trainee may be able to do 3 days a week of interval training, whereas a more advanced one may be able to do only 1 or 2 days a week or none at all.

Adaptations to your training are a consolidation of imposed stressors, which determine your muscle gains, fat loss, and strength level. Learn to spot the signs of poor recovery because some days, it's not only OK but also beneficial to take a break and just breathe but you are going to have to evaluate that according to how you are feeling and your own life happenings.

SLEEP

We now know that sleep restriction affects several behaviors including choice and amount of food intake, but less is known about how dietary patterns affect sleep; study suggests that consuming less fiber may be one of the factors associated with lighter, less restorative sleep.

On another note, we also know that there have been many people that lost weight with restrictive diets only to regained it all back when they stopped dieting and previous habits were restored, and since it is not sustainable to live a life of restriction forever, diets don't seem to work for most people in the long run.

Instead, changing behaviors that are sustainable long-term seem to work much better. We also know that, unless you already consume lots of vegetables, adding vegetables to your daily intake can improve many health measures, and guess what else comes with more vegetables?... More fiber.

So, there, add a serving of vegetables (or two) consistently for about two months, I don't care if you blend them in your sauces or smoothies, you hide them in your burgers or meatloaf, or if you enjoy them cooked, broiled, or in a scrumptious salad, as long as you add them. As far as it concerns me, that simple behavior may be the only one ever needed and it may also improve your sleep, also, adding instead of restricting, win-win if you ask me.

https://www.ncbi.nlm.nih.gov/pubmed/26156950

Sleep restriction reduced gut hormones (PYY and GLP-1) and increased appetite sensations but did not alter EE or substrate utilization during 48-h calorimeter measurements. Moreover, a 3-night shortened sleep intervention reduced CBT for 48 h in healthy young men. Three nights of short sleep duration might lead to a positive energy balance. These findings suggest that the quantity of sleep-time leads to changes in individual energy balance and circadian rhythms and may increase the risk of obesity.

https://www.ncbi.nlm.nih.gov/labs/pmc/articles/PMC5223114/

Night Shift Workers:

Unfortunately, that's common when working night shifts but plan ahead when there is no other option.

"The effect of a disrupted sleep cycle on energy metabolism is real but of modest size. In the end, it's about the practicalities of food access, convenience, and the time demands of the shift. Planning ahead is your friend. Your first thought should be hydration—go for water and other calorie-free drinks because you will need a lot of it. Dehydration, paradoxically often from too much caffeine, is a common cause of fatigue.

"Before your shift, eat the main meal with whole grains and other complex starches to curb your hunger and cravings.

"Take your own food with you so that you don't fall into the delivery service and vending machine trap. Convenience foods typically contain extra calories, sugar, saturated fat, and salt, but do not keep you full for long. Sugary and salty foods are also a major reason for the weight gain that is such a common problem for shift workers.

"Plan for your meal breaks: high protein foods like chicken and hummus are filling and calm cravings, while prepackaged healthy snacks, such as unsalted nuts and cut vegetables, are accessible on the run. Always pack water with your lunch box."

https://www.bmj.com/content/365/bmj.l2143

Injury Recovery

INJURY RECOVERY
How the body works

Tissue damage – whether from surgery or injury –
kicks off a 3-stage recovery process.

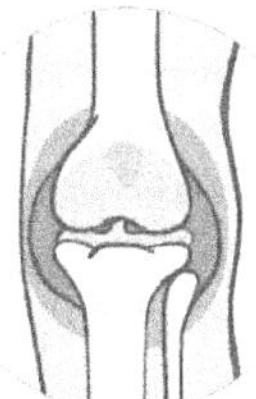 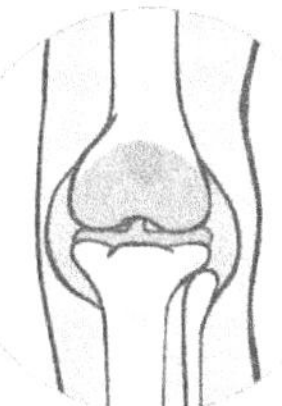 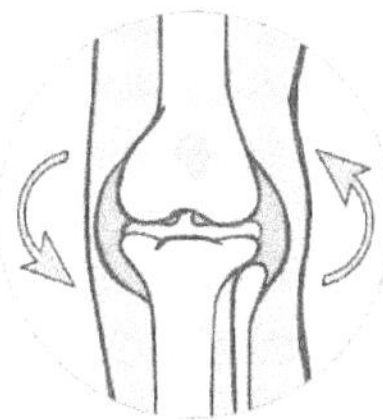

1ST STAGE: Inflammation	2ND STAGE: Proliferation	3RD STAGE: Remodeling
Pain, swelling, redness and heat; draws healing chemicals to the injured area.	Damaged tissues are removed; new blood supply and temporary tissue is built.	Stronger, more permanent tissue replaces temporary tissue.

Nutrition is extremely powerful in all three stages.

*Image Precision Nutrition

As far as the body's concerned, the ideal scenario would occur when energy intake perfectly matches energy expenditure. We also know that it will fight to stay there, and there are very important reasons for our body to try to maintain this homeostasis or 'unchanging' state.

Because energy imbalances can affect a lot more than weight gain or loss. Drastic changes in energy balance can impact other processes in the body, such as reproduction, cognitive functions, metabolic functions, repair, and regeneration.

In athletes or highly active individuals, energy deficits can impair the resynthesis of muscle and liver Glycogen, as well as the stimulation of protein synthesis. This means that our bodies don't properly repair and restore from exercise since, with a negative energy balance, the body is always functioning in a catabolic/breakdown state. With energy reserves being used to maintain a minimum level of function, there's little left over for rebuilding and repair.

In general, the macronutrients (proteins, carbohydrates, and fats), micronutrients (vitamins and minerals), and phytochemicals we eat are broken down into smaller sub-units such as amino acids, glucose, fatty acids, etc. These nutrients are taken up by our cells in particular ways, they provide potential energy, they can act as co-factors for chemical reactions in the body. They stimulate the release of hormones, and they provide raw materials that can be incorporated into our body structures, including tissues and organs.

Even though not everyone responds the same way to the digestion and absorption of specific foods, or the uptake of specific nutrients into the cell, 99.9% of people do. Recent nutritional research suggests that the basic mechanism is the same but there are intriguing individual differences likely due to our unique genetic makeup. This code provides cellular instruction for making proteins. But genetic polymorphism and nutrigenomics, though interesting, are out of the scope of this article. So, while we shouldn't eliminate food groups because they all work together synergistically, I am going to focus on the proteins we consume from food, that are synthesized into the "building blocks" for the production of 'new' proteins needed for growth and repair of tissues.

The RDA guideline for protein is 0.8 grams per kilogram of body weight per day. But athletes and lifters concerned with their performance or physique require more protein than that. And when healing from injuries, broken anything, or tissue trauma, we may need as much daily protein as recovery from heavy strength training or even more.

The researchers concluded that "…the range of 2.3 to 3.1 grams per kilogram of FFM (fat-free mass) is the most consistently protective intake against losses of lean tissue." In other words, for every kilogram of your body that's not fat, you should be consuming 2-3 grams of protein in order to preserve lean tissue.

In short, when injuries occur, we have to pay special attention to supplying our bodies with enough of these building blocks for repair. And why we often feel or hear that DOMS are worse, pain comes back, and injuries relapse while on a caloric deficit.

Whether it is tissue repair or muscle damage, our body is under stress and what happens can be summed up in three stages:

Inflammation, which draws healing chemicals to the injured area. Proliferation, which removes damaged tissues and rebuilds temporary new tissue. And remodeling, where strong more permanent tissue replaces the temporary tissue.

Until all these stages have taken place, a caloric deficit is not recommended. Remember that the goal of training is progress and adaptation, not being tired or sore, much less unrecovered completely from an injury, if there is pain, something may not be completely healed and needs a bit of special care, including rest, sleep, and proper nutrition.

To sum it up: Repair of any kind is a longer process than we might be willing to allow, but if we attempt a caloric deficit, nutrients tend to go to basics/surviving needs instead of repairing. Injuries and pain are usually felt more and heal slower. It is mainly the basic science of catabolism/anabolism. Injuries need a bit of extra protein, so make sure you add a bit more than usual to help with the healing process and wait until it is all healed up and then some before resuming activities. Remember that muscle memory is a thing and no matter how much muscle/strength you may end up losing, you'll be able to gain it back much faster than you initially gained it.

Clarifications from reader's questions:

Protein requirement is not a number set in stone, it depends on several variables including quality of protein ingested, age, fitness level, and of course, individual repair needs. The recommended minimum for sedentary individuals is 0.8g/Kg, this translates to about 55g of protein per day for a 150lb individual. However, this amount is not optimal but simply to prevent protein deficiency. During high-intensity training, these needs may be increased to about 1.4 to 2.0g per Kg of body mass (between 95 and 135g of protein per day for a 150lb individual). Similar increases are recommended during periods of low energy intake or low carbohydrate intake.

While these recommendations may be adequate to cover protein turnover requirements, research has suggested that higher amounts of protein in the diet may be vital for immune function, metabolism, satiety, weight management, and performance. Therefore, many experts recommend a higher intake that approaches or exceeds 1g of protein per pound of bodyweight.

5- Facts that may help you reach your goals easier

Good carbs, bad carbs (no such thing), and the humble potato.

We've already talked about how the food we eat is composed of a variety of nutrients. As the chemical structures of these nutrients are fairly large, we must break them down into smaller, unbound, more soluble units in order to be absorbed into the body.

Once absorbed, these smaller units become usable by our cells and once they enter the general circulation, their actual food source doesn't really matter; once broken down and absorbed, the body doesn't necessarily recognize the difference between the amino acids derived from whey protein in the form of protein powder or the ones derived from milk. Nor does it recognize the difference between glucose derived from whole wheat bread or the one from table sugar. And it doesn't recognize the difference between monounsaturated fats from a hamburger or monounsaturated fats from olive oil.

The difference is in the nutrients they deliver, so you do want some fruits and vegetables for fiber, vitamins, minerals, and phytosterols but other than that, it doesn't matter where your carbs are coming from once you met nutrition needs, that's why the 80% whole foods and 20% whatever you want works well. That said, for satiety purposes, potatoes are the single most satiating food there is.

What is NEAT?

NEAT (Non-Exercise Activity Thermogenesis) Adaptations

Probably the most significant adaptation to weight changes is in NEAT

With weight loss, your body burns fewer calories doing your usual daily chores such as pacing or fidgeting; it also decreases your motivation to conciously and subconciously move.

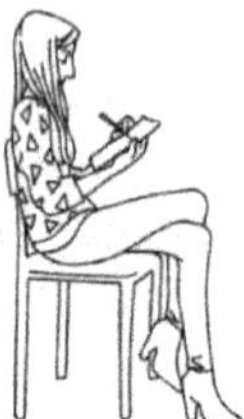
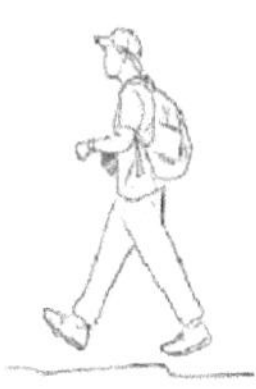
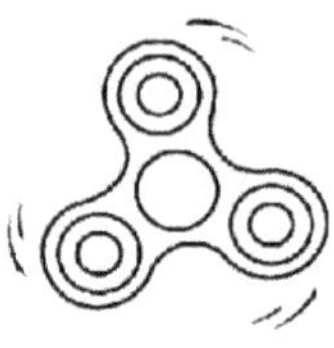

More Sitting   Less Pacing/Walking   Less Fidgeting   Less Overall Calories Burned

Breaking out with fad diets

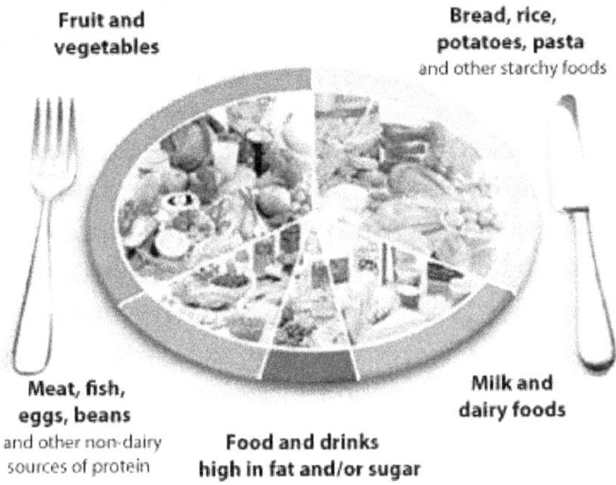

Why do so many people swear by them if they aren't as good, you ask? Well… in some cases, fad or restrictive diets seem to work in the initial phase, they even provide the dieter with some exceptional blood work for the first time (possibly not for long), and other times, they help some people instill some good habits but in most cases, these diets stop working or get people into unhealthy behaviors, illnesses, or malnutrition, if not lead them to regain the weight lost and then some. Let's explore why and what can be done about it or instead of. Because anything a fad or restrictive diet can do, a balanced diet can do better.

Over the years, one thing I've been observing in nutrition is that fad diets only become more extreme versions of themselves and are remarketed a few years later, exactly when the previous ones are being ditched because they either stopped working or they weren't sustainable and sooner or later people run into one issue or another.

Low-Carb, Atkins, Paleo, ketogenic, carnivore, snake, fasting for longer than you should, and whatever other nonsense you can imagine in between. Same with the Mediterranean, plant-based, vegetarian, vegan, whole 30, etc. Diets tend to go from moderately restrictive to plain insane for no other reason than the previous one stopped working and people don't know where to go other than a more extreme version of what seemed to work. But, more restrictive or extreme is not better or more effective, it is only more restrictive and more extreme; thus, less flexible and balanced is what it is. And they have an amazingly high failure rate in the long run.

Mind you, sometimes eliminating some food groups such as the "eating clean" crowd, leads the person to consume more whole foods that are more nutritious, and if they stop there, and they still allow some of the foods they love and don't get obsessive over "clean eating" to the point of orthorexia or deal with any restrictive/binge episodes that can send them to eating disorder territory, it may actually improve their overall nutrition profile and they can happily say, "it worked for me". The problem is that this is not always the case, and more often than not, the extreme approach does come back to haunt you in one way or another.

Most fad or restrictive diets give some initial result for weight loss, in some cases, the elimination of certain foods leads the person to eat less or fewer calories so weight loss happens. In other cases, the replacement of calorie-dense foods by nutrient-dense foods gives the person more energy, better nutrition, and a good feeling, in others, when they introduce more vegetables or more protein, they find that it leads to better overall health, all that is good in the initial phase until the extreme nonsense hits the fan. And nonsense comes when their version of the diet stops working and the person starts beating themselves up thinking they aren't dieting hard enough so they need to go more extreme, or in the worst cases, believing that there's something wrong with their metabolism.

You've listened to every guru and every opinionated individual that told you "it worked for me, you should try it" until, (what they didn't get to tell you), it stopped working or gave them an eating disorder, malnutrition, medical condition, psychological issues, etc.

And this is in no way people's fault because when you are doing the most hardcore version of one diet and you stall, the only logical thing to do is going more extreme; so that's when you go from whichever diet gave some result to the next expecting it to work better, and then the next and then... then what? Now what?! HELP!!!!

This is the point where some people finally stop and either get serious about getting professional help, sign up for coaching, or get frustrated and give up, or even worst, end up with some sort of "unknown" or unrecognized medical/metabolic/hormonal condition that some influencer is probably telling them that they can cure by… guess what? Following some other miraculous diet…

Others remain in this cycle of listening to those that had some initial result or buying into the next fad for years while yo-yo dieting and hopping from one diet to the next, I mean, there's a reason why you have so many to choose from because if they'd work for good, there wouldn't be that many more to keep choosing from.

I've worked with many people in these situations, and there was not even one time that they weren't happy to finally switch to a more moderate and balanced approach. Even if they had to be patient about it and trust the process, it may take more work on their part because it seriously involves some re-learning and habit changes, but in the end, they don't feel restricted or stuck in a vicious extreme cycle anymore.

Some people need to hit rock bottom to stop and realize that doing the same thing over and over and expecting different results won't miraculously work this time, and the more aggressive or restrictive we go, the less sustainable it is going to be. It's not your fault, it's human physiology, drastic measures are sustained by some for short periods of time but attempting them for long periods of time or forever is not only not going to happen but also not a way of living because the restrict/binge cycles aren't a fun place to be in and they do lead to eating disorder behaviors that may end up in a serious condition.

That's why fad diets, random and capricious elimination without reason, restrictions, and drastic measures that lead to more restriction and drastic measures aren't the way. There is a better way and if you think about how many years you've been spending looking for a way that didn't help then being patient and doing it right with one step at a time, maybe the way you've been looking for. One habit at a time, in a year you may be able to instill about 6 habits and end in a much better place. Stop the nonsense. There is a better way.

Fad Diets: Lifestyle Promises and Health Challenges:

Carbs; why do some people fear them and others love them?

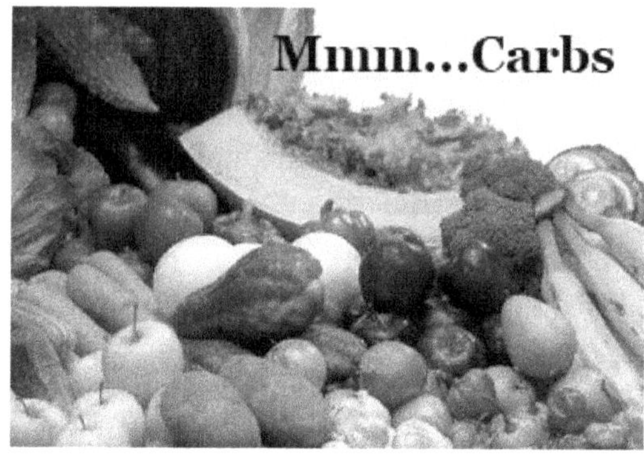

Long ago we realized that eating bread, or carbohydrates in general showed us a quick increase in scale weight, and sometimes we felt bloated and clothes seemed tighter. But now we have new knowledge that explains why it happens and why it shouldn't be a concern.

Most carbs that people tend to vilify aren't carbs but highly palatable foods combining carbs and fats plus flavorings that easily overeaten. Carbs will give you a lot more volume than fats. Fruits and vegetables are carbs. Spinach and leafy greens are great for energy and fiber.

Think about carbohydrates like they are little sponges, they absorb water, for every gram of carb you consume, our body holds onto 4 grams of water, so when you stop consuming carbs, our body starts flushing all that extra water that was bound to each gram of carbohydrate, this is the reason why some people think carbs make them fat or that keto works like magic when in reality, unless they managed a caloric deficit, it only flushes water weight that is regained the moment carbs are reintroduced.

On that note, a hydrated body performs better and carbs are a great source of energy to fuel your workouts as well as provide most of the fiber we need for health and well-being. Also, keep in mind that protein and carbs are 4 calories per gram and fats are 9 calories per gram. Fats are very caloric dense, meaning that a little miscalculation can put you over your calorie allotment quickly, and that's the main reason why at some point the ketogenic diet stops working, and adding carbs back will have to happen gradually or you'll get very bloated due to the sudden water retention, the scale will go up quickly as well but it is mostly water.

Also, did you know that protein can spike insulin as much or more than carbs? And that when meals are mixed they don't offer the same response?

Further reading:

Bonus material in our Blog:

https://strengthsisters101.com/blog/

CARBOHYDRATE CONFESSIONS:

https://www.precisionnutrition.com/low-carb-convert?
fbclid=IwAR2cG_Ue_zifPKnTt8anDsmuFiJKxrMQvQu4fXFnwx6ucwgZ
ZYsdwaDyG2A

INSULIN AN UNDESERVED BAD REPUTATION (PART I OF THE SERIES):

https://weightology.net/insulin-an-undeserved-bad-reputation/

Calories: Total Macronutrient Intake, Energy Expenditure, and Net Energy Stores.

"The energy cost of storing dietary fats as triglycerides is lower than that of converting protein or carbohydrates into fat. Donato and Hegsted (1985) have suggested that in growing animals, dietary fat can be stored as body fat with little energy expenditure and, therefore, that dietary fat stored as adipose tissue fat still yields approximately 9 kcal per gram. In contrast, energy is required to store dietary carbohydrates as body fat, and 4 kcal per gram of dietary carbohydrate yields only approximately 3.27 kcal when stored as fat and subsequently oxidized for energy. Therefore, the ratio of the energy required to store dietary fat as body fat relative to the energy cost to store dietary carbohydrates or protein as body fat may be close to 9 to 3.27. That is, the conversion of fats in food to body fat (triglycerides) is more efficient than the conversion of carbohydrates or protein in food to body fat."

https://www.ncbi.nlm.nih.gov/books/NBK218769/?fbclid=IwAR2wt7K4rCKwp6miagV2fFVZAGUlvyuw4EZLkRTj_tXRUV1tG-TrXKLpn3I

Whole vs. white bread:

THE ONLY DIFFERENCE IS THE FIBER CONTENT, SO IF YOU GET YOUR FIBER FROM OTHER SOURCES, WHITE OR WHEAT WOULD BE NO DIFFERENT:

https://examine.com/nutrition/is-whole-wheat-bread-better-than-white-bread/

Coaching available for strength, powerlifting, and nutrition at: https://strengthsisters101.com/

linktr.ee/strengthsisters101

ABOUT THE AUTHOR

Mariana Molinari-Abadie

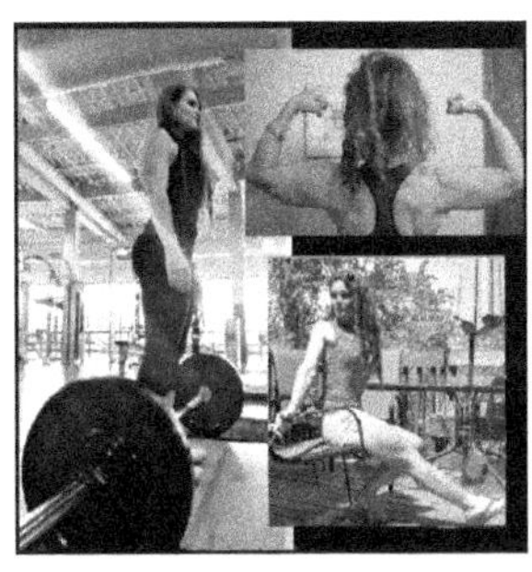

Mariana has been a teacher for many years, she loves learning and passing on knowledge, she holds many certifications from Precision Nutrition to several International Sports Sciences Association credentials as well as being a certified Powerlifting Programming Coach. Still, they don't hold a candle to the intuitive way she programs nutrition and training for her many clients both online and on the gym floor.

She has also learned from working under Registered Dietitians' mentorship and by studying nutrition science at Buenos Aires University. She loves reading research as well as consistently learning to improve her skills. She is known for asking multiple questions to ensure she has a thorough understanding, looking at the big picture, and thoroughly addressing the needs of her clients, getting them on track quickly, with ease, and in a sustainable manner.

She was born in Argentina from Italian ancestors and currently lives in the USA. She speaks multiple languages and enjoys art, reading, painting, cooking, and traveling other than lifting and getting stronger. Currently owns her own company Strength Sisters 101 along with her business partner Tanye Lacombe. Together they help people get stronger, get muscle definition, optimize their nutrition needs, fight aging and osteoporosis, feel better, and gain confidence every day.